A Spy in the Nursing Home

EILEEN KRAATZ

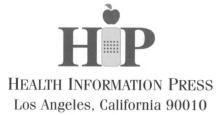

HEALTH INFORMATION PRESS
Los Angeles, California 90010

Printed in the United States of America

ISBN 1-885987-17-X

Health Information Press
a division of PMIC
4727 Wilshire Blvd., Suite 300
Los Angeles, CA 90010
(800) MED-SHOP

The information presented in this book is based on the experience and interpreta-
tion of the author. Although information has been carefully researched and
checked for accuracy, currency and completeness, neither the author nor the publisher accept any responsiblity or liability with regard to errors, omissions, mis-
use, or misinterpretation.

DEDICATION

This book is dedicated to all the dear people who reside in nursing homes. I consider each one my mother, my father. I treasure the wisdom they give to all who would take the time to listen. May those who care for their daily needs do so with the deepest respect and love.

ACKNOWLEDGMENTS

I wish to thank my husband, Chris, for his encouragement, his patience, and his steadfastness throughout the years it has taken to first experience and then to write this book. His opinions and expertise are appreciated more than he will ever know.

I thank Kathryn Swanson for her meticulous editing, her enthusiasm, and her sensitivity to the subject.

I also wish to thank Mary and Tom Spademan for their encouragement and nudging when things bogged down and time stood still.

TABLE OF CONTENTS

PREFACE

When I was seventeen, my aunt asked me to accompany her on a visit to a nursing home. I wasn't thrilled at the invitation but agreed to go anyway. That's the day I met Walter. That's the day my world burst open and revealed life as more than adolescent visions of timeless health, love, and dreams fulfilled.

Walter was my shaman, my guide, into this new world. I first spotted him sitting alone in the corner of the nursing home dining room. He wore an old blue sweater, a scarf around his neck, and cozy slippers on his feet. I approached him quietly and said, "Hi, my name's Missy, what's yours?" He lifted his head and stared right past me with black, blind eyes. After a long moment, he blessed me with the smile of Buddha. "I like the sound of your voice," he whispered.

The bond of friendship was instantly sealed in that simple exchange. We discovered that we shared the same great love of music. I was preparing to enter university as a music major. Walter had been a well-known pianist and organist until arthritis attacked his hands and froze them into fists. He'd lost his sight about the same time. We spent the whole afternoon together, an unlikely twosome: a young girl full of dreams and promise and an old man stripped of the physical ability to do what he loved the most.

At the end of our first visit, Walter placed his gnarled fist in my hand and said, "Come, I have a gift for you." Hand in hand we walked to the other side of the room where an old piano stood against the wall. Walter settled himself on the piano bench, hunched over the keyboard and placed his fists on the keys. In cruel slow motion, his fingers stretched out to form a chord and he began to play that old Scottish song, *Will Ye No Come Back Again*, asking in music the words he was too shy to speak. As the last note faded,

I put my arms around him and whispered in his ear, "See you next week, Walter."

Our weekly visits continued until Walter died. I hope I brought him joy and friendship. He gave me so much more: his wise observations about life, about facing adversities, about courage, about loneliness, about humor. But the greatest gift was the conviction that the elderly are one of our richest assets, that they are human beings to be cherished, nurtured and respected every day of their lives no matter what their physical or emotional limitations might be.

This conviction of the enduring value of our elderly—and the indifferent, sometimes abusive care I saw in Walter's nursing home—set me on my path as an advocate for better nursing home care. Over the years, I've worked as an activity director, a music therapist and as a volunteer. I've seen wonderful nursing homes and I've seen terrible ones. I passionately believe that each of us must become involved in making sure that our elderly receive the dignified and loving care they so richly deserve. Isn't that what we'd demand for ourselves and our families?

At a time when society is actively pushing for better daycare centers for our children, scrutinizing every aspect of our children's care, why do we ignore the quality of care that's given to our elderly? If we knew that a daycare center left its children in dirty diapers all day long, or restrained them in chairs, or tied their arms down, or gave them sedatives so they'd behave better, or hit them, or let them stare at television for hours, what would we do? How would society deal with the situation? You and I know the outrage such offenses would cause; the punishment the courts would dole out; the frenzy of the media coverage. Why doesn't society have the same reaction when our elderly are abused in exactly the same way in many of our nursing homes? Do we see them as so unimportant, so useless, so near the end of life that we simply choose to ignore such blatant violations of human rights?

The good news is that the media and the general public are beginning to notice and to talk about the horrors of elder abuse. But they've only scratched the surface. With the aging of the baby boomers, society's "dirty little secret" will, hopefully, be exposed and we will be as vigilant about the quality of care we give our elderly as the care we give our children. That will take time and education and commitment from all of us.

And that's the main point of this book—to alert the reader to what really goes on behind the scenes in nursing homes. Too many people think that what looks good *is* good. I continue to be amazed when someone says, "Well, the place looks clean so it must be good," or "The view from the bedrooms is just wonderful. Mom will love it here!" People tend to grasp at anything positive they see and assume it's a decent facility because they don't know what to look for and they are overwhelmed at the thought of placing a loved one in a nursing home. This is especially true when a family is in the middle of a crisis and must find a home for their loved one in a hurry. Time after time I've seen families rush into this major decision with no help and little knowledge of how or where to begin to look. All too often they end up making the wrong choice. Their loved one is unhappy and the family is miserable.

This book is written to help you avoid such a sad outcome. It guides you step by step through a difficult time and helps you collect all the information you'll need to make the right decision. The tips and tactics are gathered from my years of observation and experience of what really goes on inside a nursing home. I've written it with you and your loved one in my mind and heart. I believe that the well-being of all who reside in nursing homes will be a major issue in the twenty-first century. Only when we as consumers demand better care for the elderly and diligently monitor that care will we be assured that all nursing home residents will be treated with dignity, respect and gentleness. Each family that strives to find the best facility for their loved one makes a difference for us all. On behalf of the elderly in every nursing home, I thank you for your effort in contributing to their better care. I know my dear friend Walter would wholeheartedly agree.

INTRODUCTION

Nobody's going to put me in a nursing home. I'd rather die first!" How often have you heard those words or even said them yourself? We vow to care for Mom, Dad, or Grandma ourselves, but there comes a time when many of us must realistically face the possibility of long-term care for ourselves or for someone we love.

Caring for someone who's a victim of a major stroke, Alzheimer's disease, or brain injury can overwhelm a family emotionally, physically, and financially. Placing your loved one in a good nursing home may be best for the patient and for your family as well. But with so many nursing homes out there, how do you find the right one?

Add to that the reality of today's hectic world, where we find ourselves overwhelmed with too much to do and not enough time. Many of us are working full-time outside the home while trying to raise a family. And, as our parents age, we may be caring for them as well as our children.

In the middle of all this "busyness," what happens if Dad has a stroke that leaves him paralyzed and unable to care for himself? The hospital staff's done everything they can and want to discharge him to a nursing home. What do you do if you haven't checked one out ahead of time? Most hospitals don't give you much time to find a good one. And to make matters worse, many of the best nursing homes have waiting lists. There might not be an opening when you need it.

This book is designed to guide you quickly and calmly through a painful, bewildering time. It's written for people who haven't been able to check out nursing homes ahead of time—people who find themselves caught in a situation that doesn't give much guidance and that screams "buyer beware." This is a 5-day plan with step-by-step instructions, inside tips, questions to ask, signs to look for, and checklists to help you evaluate any nursing home.

This guide is a result of my 20 years of experience as a patients' advocate in nursing homes. Having been a paid staff member and a volunteer, I *know* what goes on behind the scenes. I know that many nursing homes look great at first glance but really aren't. Some staff members can treat residents like kings and queens when relatives visit—and hit them later. Charts can be "fixed" before state inspections. Social activities can be scheduled but never occur. The list goes on. But there are many good nursing homes out there, too. You just have to know what to look for, what questions to ask, and how to double check all answers on your own. I hope that my experience and advice will help you to be as informed as possible so that you can choose the right home with confidence.

I should mention that there are several terms for a nursing home. They include "skilled nursing facility," "extended care facility," and "skilled care facility," to name a few. But, I'll use the term "nursing home" since that's the one most of us use in daily conversations.

Just for the record, even though this book is for those who haven't the time or never thought about checking out nursing homes beforehand, it's really best to do so long before you need one. This is especially important for people who are caring for someone with Alzheimer's disease. Many good nursing homes have special staff and programs for Alzheimer's patients. You'll want to place your loved one's name on the home's waiting list well *before* you need it, and this means finding the right place while there's plenty of time.

For those who have the time, the best way to start your investigation is to work as a volunteer in the nursing home you think might be your first choice. As a volunteer, you can observe many situations discussed in this book. Since volunteer programs usually include a short training period, you would have to do this well before you need the services of the home.

Although this book is written specifically for those who suddenly must find a nursing home and haven't checked one out ahead of time, it's also very useful for anyone looking at nursing homes as a possible need in the future.

2

The first thing to remember if you need to find a facility quickly is: **DON'T PANIC!** First of all, the hospital can't just "kick" your dad out. Anyone who's covered by Medicare has the right to challenge the hospital about an early release and to stay in the hospital without paying extra costs until the case is reviewed. This can buy you some time to find a decent nursing home. You can also get help from the hospital's discharge planning staff since they can refer you to nursing homes.

Keep in mind that a referral from the hospital does *not* guarantee that the nursing home is a good one. You'll still have to check it out thoroughly. If you can afford to arrange for temporary nursing care at home, you'll find it will give you extra time to check out the nursing homes on your list. Home care may be expensive but it would be short-term and would give you peace of mind while you do your investigating.

By using this 5-day plan, you should be able to thoroughly check out any home within one week, depending on the availability of the staff for interviews. At the end of your investigation you'll know for sure whether or not it's the right place. And if the nursing home you choose has a waiting list, you may have to place your loved one in another home temporarily or use home care while you wait for the better one to become available.

The bottom line in your investigation is *loving care*. Isn't that what you really want for your mother or father or yourself? When you're doing your research ask yourself:

1. Would Mom be content living here?
2. Would Dad be kept clean and receive gentle care in this place?
3. Would I be content living here?

Ask yourself these questions *often*. If you can honestly answer "yes" to all of them, it's a pretty good bet you've found the right place.

A big factor in finding the right home is the help you receive from your friends and family members who participate in your investigation. They can help by using Checklist 2 (found at the end of Chapter Two) during a visit to the home. Please feel free to make copies of that checklist for them to use. Hopefully, they'll visit the home at different times of the day. By comparing observations, you'll get an overall picture of the home from several sources. This information will be invaluable when making your decision.

Your investigation includes 4 or 5 visits to the nursing home, using your checklists, and interviewing several staff members. The checklists appear at the end of each chapter. By reading the explanations and tips first, you'll be able to quickly check off your answers in the checklists. The checklists help keep you focused, save time, cover all aspects, and guarantee that you're asking all the right questions. The questions also show the staff that you know what to look for and you're confident in what you're doing. All of this leads to more honest answers and a clearer picture about the quality of care residents receive. With this method, you'll know you've done your homework and you'll feel good about your decision.

Chapter 1

DAY 1: BEFORE THE FIRST VISIT

It's necessary to do some ground work before you actually make your first visit to a home. This might seem tedious but you've got to know some basic facts first. The following are steps and tips, with explanations, to help you get started.

Use Checklist 1 at the end of the chapter when you begin your actual research. It lists the questions you'll want to ask.

1. Find someone who has a relative or friend in a nursing home.

Ask your friends, acquaintances, associates at work, and people in your church or synagogue (including your pastor, priest, or rabbi) if they know someone who's in a good nursing home. Ask if you can go along on their next visit. This will give you a good opportunity to begin your investigation. Ask if friends or family members who'll be helping you can also visit the same resident. This would give them a legitimate reason for going through the home. (And most residents in nursing homes love to have visitors.)

2. Keep it a secret!

Tell the person you're accompanying why you want to visit and that you'll need to spend about 2 hours at the home. Ask him or her *not* to tell anyone that you're really conducting your own investigation. You don't want to alert any of the staff about your interest in the home until you've finished this visit. I've seen it happen many times—a staff member sees someone who seems to be checking the place out, the staff member alerts the rest of the staff and they all put on a very good show! This is not always the case, but it happens often enough that you want to make sure you don't give yourself away. You want to get the *real picture* without anyone knowing what you're doing.

3. Line up a few friends or family members to visit the home at different times and days.

Let's refer to these people as "helpers" from now on. Feel free to make copies of Checklist 2 for your helpers to use during their visit. Make sure they do *not* inform anyone that they're helping with your investigation. At this point, everyone is just visiting!

4. Before you investigate any nursing home, telephone the office and ask if the facility is a Medicare- and Medicaid-certified facility.

Make sure that ALL of the rooms are certified for Medicare and Medicaid. This is important for several reasons:

- Medicare and Medicaid will not pay for care unless the home is a certified facility.
- Homes that participate in Medicare and Medicaid programs are called "certified facilities" and must meet federal standards, whereas non-certified nursing homes don't necessarily have to meet the same standards.
- Certified facilities are inspected more often than non-certified nursing homes.

- If you don't have Medicaid when you enter a nursing home that isn't certified, you can be evicted when your money and insurance run out. Medicaid-certified homes must allow you to stay and must accept Medicaid payments when you qualify.

- If you choose a home that has a limited number of rooms certified for Medicare or Medicaid, you can only get those benefits if you stay in a certified room. And sometimes rooms get changed! Do your homework. It's only a telephone call but it's crucial!

Nursing home care is expensive. The average cost for private-paying residents is about $36,000 a year. Therefore, you want to find out as much as you can about the expenses, what coverage you or your loved one has (whether it's Medicare, Medicaid, or a private insurance plan), and what the personal cost will be.

5. Find out about Medicare.

Medicare is a national health insurance program. It's divided into two parts: Part A helps pay for hospital care and nursing home care while Part B helps pay various other bills like doctor bills and other medical service fees. If you or your spouse are 65 years old, have held a Medicare-covered job for at least 10 years, and are a citizen or permanent resident of the United States, you are eligible for Part A of Medicare without having to pay any premium for it. This is also true if you're receiving Social Security or Railroad Retirement benefits or if you're eligible but haven't signed up for those benefits yet. You can also receive Part A if you're receiving kidney dialysis or if you're a kidney transplant patient.

Please be aware that Medicare only covers the first 100 days of a stay in a nursing home, and to receive it you must have been in the hospital for at least 3 consecutive days prior to entering a home. For the first 20 days all expenses are covered, but then the coverage goes down and Medicare only pays a portion of the cost (you pay up to $95.50 per day). On the 101st day, you must pay all costs for the rest of the stay.

To obtain Part B of Medicare, which does NOT cover nursing home care, you must pay a monthly premium. In 1998, the monthly premium for Part B was $43.80 with a $100 yearly deductible. For further information on Medicare, I strongly urge you to call the Social Security Administration. Their toll-free number is 1-800-772-1213.

An excellent source of information on Medicare is *Medicare and You.* You can get this handbook by sending a request to:

Health Care Financing Administration
7500 Security Blvd.
Baltimore, MD 21244-1850

The handbook is also available on audio tape and on the Internet. The web site is http://www.hcfa.gov

Another helpful book is *Medicare Made Simple,* by Denise Knaus. It can be obtained at your local bookstore, or by calling the publisher directly at 1-800-MED-SHOP. Other books are listed in Appendix B at the back of this book.

6. Call your state's Office on Aging, or your state's Department of Social Services for information on Medicaid.

Do this as soon as you begin to consider anything about nursing homes. You must know what your state requires and what financial help it provides. Medicaid for nursing home care is available for people with low incomes and for nursing home residents who have spent all their resources on care. People who are on Medicaid are protected by a Federal law that requires Medicare/Medicaid-approved nursing homes to provide room and board and basic daily care. This includes meals, a semi-private room, nursing care, basic grooming care, some dental care, social services, and activities. Medicaid also pays for other basic needs like incontinence supplies, soap, toothpaste, razors, laundry, etc. It's important that you check this out at your state's Department of Social Services. They'll help you determine your eligibility.

You must meet certain requirements to be eligible for Medicaid, and you must also be assessed to see if you need nursing home care. States vary on this and you should find out what's required where you live. In most states, your assets must be lower than $2,000. This does not include your house, or car or personal belongings. If you're married, your spouse retains your home and income of at least $1,870 per month as well as at least $14,964 in liquid assets or resources and your home.

7. If you're in a hurry...

Ask the Office on Aging or Department of Social Services to send you the information as quickly as possible (preferably by overnight express), or ask them if there's a place in your city where you can pick up the information.

8. If the person entering a nursing home has a private long-term care insurance policy, READ THE FINE PRINT!

Please be sure to go over this with a lawyer or insurance representative. These policies vary in their coverage and you want to know exactly what the one you'll be using does and does not cover. Nursing homes can bill a private-paying resident for many services. Over and above the daily rate for room and board and basic care, they can charge you for extras such as dental care, special therapy, and even wheelchairs. The list can seem endless. Private insurance also varies in the amount of money paid out and the length of time covered. If the insurance plan is not adequate for your loved one's needs, he or she could end up using all his or her savings and still have to go on Medicaid. It's extremely important that you find out **exactly** what that policy covers.

9. Don't assume that a church-sponsored facility is a good one.

It's no guarantee. One of the worst homes I worked in was affiliated with a mainline Christian denomination. Again, *do your own checking!*

10. Some states allow small homes to care for 6 residents with only one staff member at all times!

This one staff member is responsible for all the cooking, cleaning, and total care of the 6 residents! Clearly, you want to avoid this kind of situation.

11. For readers who live in Canada, please note that the provincial governments are responsible for overseeing all aspects of nursing home care.

This includes certification, inspections, medical coverage and eligibility. Because each province has its own standards and requirements, you must call your provincial Ministry of Health listed in your local telephone directory. For general information, you can also call the Ministry of Health in Ottawa at (613) 957-2991 or (613) 954-8616. Be sure to obtain all the financial information you can. Ask the same questions listed for Medicare and Medicaid. Find out where you can get the information locally, or request your provincial Ministry of Health to sent it by overnight express mail.

CHECKLIST FOR DAY 1: Before the First Visit

The following are the steps you should cover and the questions you should ask before your first visit:

1. Name of the nursing home:

2. Name of person who has a relative or friend in the nursing home:

3. Name of resident you will be visiting:

4. Day and time of first visit:

5. Is the home a Medicare/Medicaid-certified facility? (Call the administrative office of the home and ask.)

   Yes_____ No_____

6. Are ALL the rooms in the facility certified for Medicare and Medicaid?

   Yes_____ No_____

7. Did you call your state Office on Aging or state Medicaid Office (or provincial Ministry of Health in Canada) for financial information?

   Yes_____ No_____

8. When and where can you get printed information?

9. Names of friends and family members who will be helping with your investigation:

Chapter 2

DAY 2: THE FIRST VISIT

The first visit to any nursing home can be a bit scary since most people don't know what to expect. But this visit is probably the most important part of your investigation. It will give you an overall picture of the quality of care your loved one will receive. The two most important things a good nursing home provides are *personal dignity* and *loving care*. You can't have one without the other. When these two qualities dominate all aspects of care, you've found an excellent nursing home. Unfortunately, in a lot of homes the residents are treated like bothersome children by overworked, underpaid, and unmotivated staff. This sort of treatment shows itself in many ways. For this reason, please be sure to use Checklist 2 at the end of this chapter. It guides you through the visit, tells you what to look for and what questions to ask.

Since the well-being of your loved one depends mainly on the care of the nursing staff, checking them out is crucial. Unless you live or work in the nursing home, you really *don't* know what goes on behind the scenes. On the surface the care may look great, but you must look deeper before you make your decision.

Looking deeper involves checking the three different shifts of nursing staff. The first shift is usually from 7:00 a.m. to 3:00 p.m., the second from 3:00 p.m. to 11:00 p.m., and the third from 11:00 p.m. to 7:00 a.m. You'll also want your helpers to check at least the first two shifts. Make copies of Checklist 2 for them to use; you'll be comparing notes and observations later. The more people who are involved in your investigation, the better you'll feel about your decision.

Listed below are some of the most common signs that tell you if the care is **not** good. Make sure that you *really look* for these because they may indicate major problems in a nursing home. The administrative and nursing staff might give you all kinds of explanations for why a certain condition is "perfectly normal" and "done all the time." **DON'T BELIEVE IT!** A breach of any of the following points makes the home unacceptable.

1. State inspection report posted.

The first thing to look for when you enter a nursing home is the latest state inspection report. Facilities approved by Medicare and Medicaid must display it in a prominent place for everyone to see. Read it and check the date. Is it current?

2. Resident's Bill of Rights posted.

The next thing to look for is a copy of the Resident's Bill of Rights (sometimes called the Patient's Bill of Rights). This should be displayed in the front lobby. It should be in large print and very visible to everyone. There should also be a copy in a prominent place on every floor of the nursing home and in every resident's room. If it isn't, **be suspicious**!

At the end of the book you'll find a condensed version of a Resident's Bill of Rights. Keep in mind that each state has its own regulations and that this is only a sample. Many nursing homes have a condensed version in large print hanging in the dining room and in each resident's room. But, think of this: If the residents have poor eyesight or physiological problems and can't read or understand the Bill, *what good is it?!* The Bill is only as good as the staff that honors it. It's sad that many residents who would like to refer to the Bill can't. They aren't strong enough to stand up for their rights, and many of them fear reprisal from the staff. That's why it's so important to find a good, caring staff—from maintenance to administration—for your loved one and for your peace of mind.

3. Use your nose.

Is there an unpleasant odor or strong disinfectant smell? As in your own home, a bad odor usually means a housekeeping problem. A good nursing home doesn't have *any* strong odor. There's *no excuse* for any hall or room smelling like a latrine! Administrators and nursing staff may tell you that all nursing homes smell like that. *It's not true.* Good maintenance can take care of any unpleasant odors and you should not accept anything less.

4. Are the residents tied in wheelchairs or geriatric chairs?

Look to see if there are a lot of residents tied in wheelchairs or geriatric chairs. Sometimes it's necessary to restrain a resident if he or she is extremely disoriented or confused. But some busy staffs will tie up residents just because they don't have time to care for their immediate needs. If you see a lot of residents in restraints, it's a warning sign.

5. Do the residents have bruises?

Pay attention to any bruises you see on residents. Many elderly people tend to bruise easily. However, if several residents are bruised, especially on the face and arms, it's a red flag. Some staff members lose control and hit a resident who is stubborn or slow. Again, ask questions and observe!

6. Are the residents sitting comfortably in their chairs or beds?

Sometimes staffs get so busy that they don't change the position of those who are slumped uncomfortably in wheelchairs, geriatric chairs or beds. Check the residents' positions at the beginning and end of your visit.

Are they still in the same uncomfortable positions or has the staff been attentive enough to make them comfortable?

7. Are the residents up and dressed?

Or are they still in their bed clothes lounging around with nothing to do?

8. Check out the general grooming of the residents.

Do their clothes look clean? Is their hair combed and clean? Are the male residents clean-shaven?

9. Are the residents wearing bibs?

Look to see if the residents are wearing bibs. In many nursing homes the residents have to wear bibs when eating, and in some homes they must wear them all day long. I think this common practice is demeaning. However, if bibs are worn all day, check to see if they're clean. When you see breakfast, lunch, or dinner crumbs on the residents' bibs and faces, the rest of their personal care won't be much better.

10. Are the incontinent residents all kept in the same common room during the day?

I've worked in homes where this is done without regard for the mental or emotional condition of the residents. Many of them may be incontinent, but they haven't lost the ability to think clearly or to enjoy the companionship of others. They don't need to be hidden away. This is often done to keep visitors from seeing or smelling anything unpleasant. It's also done when the housekeeping staff doesn't clean frequently enough.

11. Are residents given privacy during bathing or toileting?

Look to see if the residents are given privacy during bathing and toileting. Many nursing homes have large tubs or showers off the main halls. Often, busy staff members don't bother to shut the door or draw the curtain while they bathe residents in full view of anyone passing by.

12. Are bedridden residents given privacy?

Look to see if the bedridden residents are given privacy. Many homes leave the bedroom doors wide open. Anyone can walk into a room without knocking. If no screens are used to protect residents' privacy, their dignity is stripped away. Many of these residents can't speak or communicate in any way. Imagine being completely helpless and totally naked for everyone to see! Of course, the staff must have doors open to keep watch over these residents, but they must also protect the dignity of even the most helpless.

13. Walk through the area where bedridden residents live.

You can't afford to be squeamish when investigating for cleanliness and quality of care. Check to see if any residents are lying or sitting in their own excrement. Friday morning is a good day to check this out. Many nursing homes give residents suppositories or enemas on Fridays so the staff won't be bothered with residents' bowel problems over the weekends. Take a mental note of what you see and then tour the rest of the home.

Return to the bedridden area at the end of your visit. Check to see how many residents are still waiting to be cleaned. It may be an unpleasant experience for you, but it's invaluable in helping to assess the facility and its staff.

14. Is the nursing staff big enough to take care of all the residents?

There should be *at least* one registered nurse (RN) (preferably) or licensed practical nurse (LPN) on duty at all times, night and day, seven days a week. There should be sufficient LPNs and aides at all times as well. If the staff is too small, the person you care about won't get the care he or she deserves.

15. Ask an aide if there's a registered nurse or licensed practical nurse on duty during your visit.

Get your helpers to do the same when they're checking out the different shifts. You'll be comparing your observations with the administrator's answer later.

16. Do the aides promptly respond to the needs of the residents?

It's very important to check out the nursing aides. They're responsible for much of the daily care and they're often much closer to the residents. They usually work the same shifts as the nurses. Watch for clues like residents sitting or lying in uncomfortable positions throughout your visit, residents calling repeatedly for help, or unanswered call buttons (there is often a light outside residents' rooms that goes on when the button is pushed). These are warning signs that there aren't enough aides or that they just don't answer promptly. These signs should tell you to take a second look at the place.

17. Look to see if any nursing staff (especially the aides) are just sitting in a resident's room or in the common room watching television.

This often happens when the daily "soaps" are on. Of course this takes the staff away from attending to the needs of the residents.

18. Listen to the tone of voice the staff uses when talking to residents.

Listen to the words they use as well. I've heard aides and nurses scream at residents, insult them, and even call them names. This is emotional and verbal abuse.

19. Observe the residents' reactions to different staff members.

You want to see warm, natural responses. This includes their reactions to nurses, aides, and maintenance personnel. Take careful note of these reactions—good and bad—because they're important clues as to how the residents are treated.

20. Talk with the residents.

Extra information can come from the residents themselves. It's important that you get their feedback. Use as many extra "eyes" and "ears" as you can! Ask them questions. Ask about the staff; ask if they have a favorite nurse; ask if they are content in the home. Don't push for answers. If the home has problems, many residents are reluctant to talk about them because they fear reprisal. Watch their body language and facial expressions in response to your questions. Be sensitive to their needs but take special note of all that's communicated, verbal and non-verbal.

21. When you're visiting a resident in his or her room, push the help button.

Wait to see how long it takes the staff to answer the bell. When the nurse or aide arrives, don't feel you need to give an explanation. Something like, "Sorry, I must have hit the wrong button," will be sufficient.

And don't let this detective work bother you. Keep in mind that you're checking the home for someone you love, and you want to make sure the care is the best that it can be. You don't want the person you love to be forced to wait one or two hours after pressing the bell. That bell is a crucial part of his or her security and care.

22. Is the call button within the resident's reach?

That button isn't any good if the resident can't reach it. This is especially true for those who are bedridden or in wheelchairs.

23. Check the bathroom of the person you're visiting.

Does it have a call button that's accessible?

24. Check the maintenance staff by observing their interaction with the residents.

Many people are involved in caring for residents and each one has an effect on their well-being. This includes the maintenance personnel since they have direct, daily contact with residents. Do they treat the residents with respect? Do they keep the rooms neat and clean? Observation is important. I once saw a maintenance man kick a blind, elderly woman who was sitting alone in her wheelchair in the dining room. This is just one example of the abuse that can happen. Please be sure to *observe, observe, observe!*

25. If you like what you've observed about the home, set up an appointment to interview the home's administrator.

At the end of your visit, stop at the administration office. Tell them that you're interested in the home and would like to make an appointment with the administrator as soon as possible. Some homes insist that you meet with the admissions coordinator instead. If you can't talk them into giving you an appointment with the administrator, and if you like the home, go ahead and make the appointment with the admissions coordinator. You'll find that I've included tips for this interview in the Day 3 section of the book, but you don't need to worry about that now.

26. While in the office, make appointments to meet with the social service director, the activity director, and the dietitian.

If possible, these meetings should come *after* your interview with the administrator. I strongly suggest this so that those whom you interview won't be able to "tip off" the administrator that you're sharp and you're asking a lot of good questions. Try to line up the administrator's interview for Day 3 and the other interviews for Day 4. This will give you the time you need to do the interviews well and not pack too much into one day. Interviews with the social service director, activity director, and dietitian won't take long. Try to line them up one after the other to save yourself from making extra trips.

Incidentally, many nursing homes hire a social service director on a consultant basis from outside the home. If the home has more than 120 beds, it *must* have a full-time social service director on its staff. If the home you're investigating is smaller than 120 beds and doesn't have a full-time social service director, you may have a bit of trouble getting an interview quickly. You'll just have to schedule it as soon as possible.

27. While in the office, ask for a copy of the Resident's Bill of Rights.

You'll want to read this in your spare time. If you have any questions concerning it, you can jot them down and ask the administrator during your interview.

28. Ask a pastor, priest or rabbi to accompany you on a surprise visit to the facility.

Have him or her wear a clerical collar or something that identifies him or her as a member of the clergy. You'd be surprised how much easier and more complete your inspection will be! Staffs let clergy go where other visitors aren't allowed.

29. Don't let this long list of tips intimidate you!

What you've just read is an in-depth explanation of why you'll be checking each of these points out. Checklist 2 puts them into simple yes/no questions to help you make your observations quickly and easily.

CHECKLIST FOR DAY 2: The First Visit

Be sure to make copies of this list for your helpers to use on their visits. Helpers should go at different times and during different shifts.

This is probably the most important checklist for your investigation. Much of it involves checking out the nursing care that residents receive. The nursing staff, which includes registered nurses (RNs), licensed practical nurses (LPNs), and nursing aides, is responsible for the daily care and well-being of your loved one. A good nursing staff can bring comfort and contentment to residents' lives. A poor nursing staff can make life miserable and cause physical and emotional decline for residents. That's why it's necessary for you to check out at least the first two shifts (and the third one if possible).

Your helpers should visit the home at different times of the day and use copies of this checklist during their investigations. The shift times are usually 7:00 a.m. to 3:00 p.m., 3:00 p.m. to 11:00 p.m., and 11:00 p.m. to 7:00 a.m. By using the following questions, you and your helpers should be able to get a good idea of the quality of the nursing staff and the overall care of the residents.

Please remember—*Don't* tell any staff member that you might be interested in the home for your loved one or for yourself. By not telling anyone, you'll help ensure that your first impression of the home is more accurate. Remind the person you're accompanying not to mention this either.

1. Do you see the latest state inspection report in a prominent spot?

    Yes_____ No_____

2. What is the date on it?_____

3. Do you see the Resident's Bill of Rights prominently displayed?

    Yes_____ No_____

4. Is it in large print? Yes_____ No_____

5. Do you see a copy of it on every floor and in the residents' rooms?

Yes_____ No_____

6. Is there an unpleasant odor in the home? Can you smell urine or a strong disinfectant?

Yes_____ No_____

7. Are there a lot of residents tied or restrained in wheelchairs or geriatric chairs?

Yes_____ No_____

8. Do you see bruises on several patients' arms or faces?

Yes_____ No_____

9. Do the residents look comfortable in their chairs or beds?

Yes_____ No_____

10. Are the residents up and dressed or still in their bedclothes?

Up and dressed_____ Not up and dressed_____

11. Are the residents' clothes clean?

Yes_____ No_____

12. Is their hair combed and clean?

Yes_____ No_____

13. Are the male residents clean-shaven?

Yes_____ No_____

14. Are the residents wearing bibs?

Yes_____ No_____

15. If so, are the bibs clean?

Yes_____ No_____

16. Are the incontinent residents grouped together in the same day room by themselves?

Yes_____ No_____

17. Does the staff help residents with grooming, toileting or bathing in private?

Yes_____ No_____

18. Do the bedridden residents have privacy? Does the staff pull curtains, use screens or shut the door when attending to these residents' needs?

Yes_____ No_____

19. Do the bedridden residents look clean and well-groomed?

Yes_____ No_____

20. Are the bedridden residents lying in their own excrement or urine?

Yes_____ No_____

21. Do you think there are enough nursing staff members (nurses, LPNs, aides) for the number of residents you see?

Yes_____ No_____

22. Did you ask an aide if there's an RN or LPN on duty during the time of your visit?

Yes_____ No_____

23. Do you see many call lights (outside residents' rooms) flashing or lit up and not being answered?

Yes_____ No_____

24. Do you hear residents calling for help?

Yes_____ No_____

25. Do you see any nursing staff (including aides) watching television in the day room or in residents' rooms instead of caring for the residents?

Yes_____ No_____

26. Do the members of the nursing staff speak respectfully to the residents?

Yes_____ No_____

27. Did you hear any verbal abuse, including unpleasant tone of voice, screaming, or name-calling?

Yes_____ No_____

28. Do you see warm, friendly interaction between residents and staff?

Yes_____ No_____

29. Did you chat with residents about the staff, a favorite nurse, things they like about the home, etc.?

Yes_____ No_____

Positive comments from residents:

Negative comments from residents:

30. Did you push the button in the room of the resident you're visiting? If so, did it take long for a staff member to respond?

Yes_____ No_____

31. Is the resident's call button within easy reach?

Yes_____ No_____

32. Does the resident's bathroom have a call button within easy reach?

Yes_____ No_____

33. Does the maintenance staff (those who clean residents' rooms, dining room, front lobby, etc.) treat residents with respect?

Yes_____ No_____

34. Go back to check the positions of residents who looked uncomfortable in their beds or chairs. Have they been made comfortable?

Yes_____ No_____

35. Go back to check any bedridden residents who were lying in their own excrement. Have they been cleaned up?

Yes_____ No_____

36. Were you able to take another quick visit with a pastor or rabbi?

Yes_____ No_____

37. If so, did you see things you hadn't seen before? Describe:

Positive:

Negative:

38. When your helpers have completed their visit with this checklist, please be sure to compare notes, perhaps over coffee or by telephone.

Chapter 3

DAY 3: INTERVIEWING THE ADMINISTRATOR

A good administrator is *crucial* to the well-being of your loved one. A good administrator knows the staff well and, ideally, knows each resident by name. He or she should be *very* visible in the nursing home and available to all residents and staff.

In many nursing homes, the first person you'll meet with is the admissions coordinator. Although this person can give you the initial information and tour, try your best to get an interview with the administrator instead. After all, the administrator is the one ultimately responsible for the care of your loved one and you have the right to an interview.

The checklist for this interview is at the end of this chapter. *Please be sure to make an extra copy of it.* You'll also find a letter to the administrator. Take the letter and two copies of the checklist to this interview because you may run into a problem and you'll have to decide what's best in your situation. Here's the potential problem: Let's say the office staff tells you that you can't interview the administrator. Ask "Why not?" If the answer is "He's too busy," or "She just doesn't interview everybody who's interested in the place," or "He just doesn't do that," etc., I'd forget the place. However, if the administrator agrees to meet with you but isn't available for another week and you're in a hurry, use the following strategy:

No matter whom you're interviewing, use the checklist.

If you can't get an interview with the administrator and you decide to go ahead and interview the admissions coordinator, use the checklist, ask the questions, write down the answers, and *keep that copy!*

Leave the letter and the extra checklist for the administrator to read, fill in, and *sign* as soon as possible. That way you'll still get his or her answers and you can compare them with those from the admissions coordinator.

If you are able to interview the administrator, take the extra copy of the checklist and the letter anyway. Emergency meetings do come up and the administrator might not be available as planned. If this happens, just leave the letter and checklist for him or her to read, fill in, and *sign*. You can pick the answers up later.

Whether you're interviewing the administrator or admissions coordinator, simply go right down the checklist and ask each question. Be sure to write down the answers. And remember, asking questions doesn't guarantee you'll get truthful answers. Ask them anyway because you'll be double checking them with your own observations. A good administrator will expect these questions and will be happy to answer them. The following list contains all the questions along with extra information for you to read before the interview (the checklist itself contains only the questions):

1. Ask the administrator if he or she has a current state license, and ask to see it.

Ask about his or her training and experience. How long has he or she been an administrator? It's important to have an experienced administrator in charge of the facility.

2. Ask to see the home's license.

Check the date of the last inspection. If the home isn't licensed or if you aren't allowed to see the license, *leave* and don't bother checking the place out.

3. Ask to see the results of the latest state inspection.

Every nursing home must be inspected by the state each year. The number and type of inspections differ from state to state. Don't feel totally secure about these reports or the ratings given by the state. Nursing homes are often notified about the inspections long before they're actually done. This gives the staff plenty of time to "clean up their act." I've seen this happen many times. Residents' records are updated, painting is done, general maintenance is upgraded, new activities are scheduled, and staffs are told to be on their best behavior. After the inspection, the old routine sets in and things just coast for another year. So read the latest state results but *do your own inspection as well.*

4. Does the home accept residents already on Medicaid?

Many nursing homes take private-paying residents before they'll take those on Medicaid because they can charge the private-paying residents more.

5. What's the home's policy for residents on Medicare?

Some give preference to those on Medicare over those on Medicaid since Medicare pays a higher rate than Medicaid. But Medicare only lasts a few weeks and many nursing homes try to discharge or transfer residents when their Medicare runs out. You must find out the home's policy on Medicare patients and *get it in writing.*

6. Does the home have a "Bed Hold" policy?

If a resident is transferred temporarily to a hospital, you must know whether or not the nursing home will hold the bed for that resident. Nursing homes charge for this. Medicaid pays to hold the bed for a short time; Medicare does *not*. Private-paying residents usually have to pay the full daily rate to have the bed held in their absence. Be sure to check the home's policy on this.

7. Ask if the home has a special unit for people with Alzheimer's disease or other types of dementia.

Many homes provide this and it sounds great, but be aware that many special units aren't well run; they're just a wing or floor where residents suffering from dementia are segregated from other residents with no special services provided. A good special unit will have specifically trained staff and activities for these residents. Be sure to tour this section if the home has one. Observe the residents. Are they just sitting around or wandering aimlessly? Ask the staff on the special unit about their training and about activities. If your loved one might be placed in the unit, check it out further by repeat visits at different times of the day.

8. Ask the administrator for the names of the staff doctors. Write them down.

It's very important that you ask the administrator about the staff doctors and then do your own checking. Too often the doctors who care for the residents aren't the best qualified. Most nursing homes don't have a doctor in residence. The doctors are on call but generally don't visit the home every day. If the home is serviced by only one or two doctors, the medical care might be minimal. Although most doctors are competent, keep in mind that there are those with questionable ability who get most of their patient load from nursing homes.

After your interviews and tours, call the local hospitals and ask for those doctors' credentials. You'll find a checklist for this purpose at the end of this chapter. Find out where they went to undergraduate school and to medical school. Ask what their specialties are. If none of the hospitals in the area have the doctors on staff, *forget* that nursing home unless you can be guaranteed that you'll have your *own* doctor.

9. Ask the administrator the following questions about the staff doctors:

- How often does each doctor visit the home?
- Is the doctor accessible?
- Is the doctor's name and telephone number given to the resident and the family?
- Who takes care of the residents when the doctor isn't available?
- Are the relatives notified immediately when there's a change in the resident's condition?

10. Does the home allow a resident to choose his or her own physician whether or not that physician is on the staff?

If it isn't allowed, *think twice* about the place.

11. Is the director of nursing a registered nurse (RN)?

The director of nursing oversees all the nursing staff. He or she is responsible for all aspects of the nursing care of the residents. A degree as a registered nurse is crucial for this position.

12. Is there at least one registered nurse (RN) or licensed practical nurse (LPN) on duty at *all* times, night and day, seven days a week?

This is a must! Ask the administrator about this and then compare his or her answer to the one you got during your first inspection on Day 2. If the home doesn't provide this, *forget the place*!

13. Ask the administrator what the ratio of nurses to residents is.

Write down the answer because you'll want to check it with your own observations.

14. Does the home use temporary staff hired from outside agencies?

Be wary of this since temporary staff members aren't familiar with the residents and their specific needs. Residents like to have the same group of people caring for them. They can become confused and upset when they don't have familiar faces helping in their daily routine.

15. Does the home provide physical, occupational, and speech therapies?

Who gives them? How often and how long are they given? Many times when residents are placed in a home, their therapy stops; or it only lasts a little while and isn't consistent. Ask about the home's policy on this and *take notes*.

16. What arrangements are there for dental, hearing, and vision care?

I know of a nursing home that arranged to have all the residents' teeth pulled so the staff wouldn't have to bother making sure they brushed their teeth! Some nursing homes don't encourage residents to wear their hearing aids or dentures, and don't bother to keep eyeglasses clean. Proper use of these is necessary for residents to communicate, to eat, and to enjoy the companionship of others. And by the way, many staffs don't bother to check hearing aid batteries or replace them.

17. Does the home have a full-time social service director?

Remember that a home with more than 120 beds must have its own full-time social service director on staff. If the home has less than 120 beds, it can have a social service director on a consultant basis.

18. Is the social service director also responsible for the activities?

If this is the case, I strongly suggest that you forget this facility. Both the social service director and the activity director are very important positions that require full attention. One person **can't** do both jobs well. The residents are the ones to suffer.

19. Ask if the home has a full-time activity director.

It's a full-time job to plan and provide enough activities to keep the residents as active, involved and happy as possible. Again, I'd forget the place if the home doesn't have one.

20. Ask to see a list of any rules residents must follow.

Do you think they're reasonable?

21. Does the home have a Resident Council?

This is a program that gives residents an opportunity to voice opinions and complaints and to have some influence on programs and policies of the home. Good nursing homes will have one of these. Ask about any recent suggestions from the Resident Council.

22. Are family members allowed to attend the Resident Council meetings?

Does the home have a Family Council as well? Family members should be allowed to voice opinions, complaints, and suggestions too.

23. Check the visitation policy of the home.

You should be able to visit any time—day or evening. There should be no limitations on visits by family members.

24. Ask about the local law and fire code for emergencies.

Watch and listen to the administrator carefully. You want to see that he or she knows the answer immediately and doesn't have to look it up.

25. Ask about staff training for emergencies like fire.

Ask how many fire drills are held each year. Is there a working sprinkler system as well as fire extinguishers? What does the local law or fire code require about sprinklers and extinguishers?

26. Are there extra charges for services that aren't included in the basic daily rate?

Many homes charge extra if residents are confused or incontinent. Other hidden charges may be added for laundry services, physical therapy, special diets, and other services that you assumed would be included. This is especially true when the resident is paying privately. Remember that nursing homes are *not* allowed to charge Medicaid residents extra for basic items and services. If there are additional expenses, how much? Ask the administrator if you can get a list of the extra charges from the administration office. *Be sure to get them in writing*!

27. Ask how the home handles residents' money.

If a resident gives written authorization, the home must handle the money for the resident and give the resident quarterly statements. Money over $50.00 must be put in an interest bearing account. If the resident is on Medicaid, the home must tell him or her when the account is getting close to the maximum allowed by Medicaid. This way, the resident can spend it before he or she loses Medicaid eligibility. This is a great law. I've been in nursing homes where the residents didn't know how much money they had and didn't know they had a right to know! This can rob a person of dignity and self-esteem. Residents need to know about their finances, whether they choose to handle them by themselves or not.

28. Does the home provide beauty and barber services?

Proper grooming is important in maintaining the dignity of the residents. Like all of us, they feel better and their self-esteem is higher when they know they're well-groomed.

29. Are there any restrictions on making or receiving telephone calls?

This right is often denied, leaving residents feeling like prisoners in the nursing home and cut off from those they love. There should be a phone available in their rooms or in a convenient place close to their rooms.

30. Are residents allowed to have their own radio and television in their room as well as a favorite chair, etc.?

This makes the place feel more like home and helps residents feel they still have some control over their lives.

31. Ask for a copy of the admission agreement.

This is a contract that tells you the services the home provides, your rights and responsibilities, the daily room rate, and all charges for care. An admission contract is quite long and contains a lot of legal terms. You need time to read it and I strongly urge you to take it to your attorney before you or your loved one signs it. Some contracts have illegal requirements such as charging pre-admission fees to people covered by Medicare or Medicaid. Get a copy and take it to a lawyer.

32. Show the administrator your checklist in which you've written his or her answers and ask if he or she would be willing to sign it.

This should include statements he or she made about the care, visitation, financing, etc. of the facility. This is *very* important. You could offer to run off a copy in the administration office and leave it (if necessary) for the administrator to read before signing. I wouldn't do this unless you sense hesitancy from the administrator. *Keep the original—don't let it out of your hands!!* Don't give it to anyone else to copy; make the copy yourself! If the administrator won't sign it, forget the place. Any statement an administrator makes while trying to interest you in a facility should be in writing and *signed*. If he or she refuses, you can be pretty sure some of the statements aren't true.

33. Ask the administrator to personally give you a tour of the home.

Hopefully, he or she will take the extra time to do this. You can't check the administrator thoroughly without being able to watch how he or she relates to staff and residents. You want to see natural, friendly reactions on their faces. Watch to see if everyone is overly friendly or "putting on a good front" for you. This happens when staff members sense the administrator is trying to "sell" the home to a potential client.

34. At the end of the tour, ask if you can visit around the place by yourself.

Sometimes, administrators or other staff members will only take you to see the nicest sections of the home, areas that are the cleanest and have the most staff. With this question, you're really testing to see how open the administrator is. Since you've already visited on Day 2, this visit will serve to double check your initial reactions to the home.

35. Use the checklist for Day 3 carefully.

Be sure to make an extra copy of this checklist and take it along with the Letter to the Administrator. That way you're prepared to leave the questions and letter in case the administrator isn't available at the last minute. Remember that if you interview the admissions coordinator, leave the letter and the extra checklist for the administrator.

If you're interviewing the administrator, *write down all answers you're given*. Take the checklist with you on a clip board or as it is in the book, and *don't be embarrassed* about asking these questions. A good administrator expects questions like these and appreciates a well-organized interview. Ask each question and don't be intimidated. Wait until the end of the interview to ask the administrator to sign your copy.

If the administrator is not available and you end up interviewing the admissions coordinator instead, *write down* all his or her answers. You'll be comparing them with the answers you get from the administrator's copy, which you'll leave for him or her to fill in.

Remember: *DON'T LET YOUR ORIGINAL COPY OUT OF YOUR HANDS!!*

CHECKLIST FOR DAY 3:
Questions for the Administrator

1. Does the administrator have a current state license?

Yes_____ No_____

2. Will he or she show it to you?

Yes_____ No_____

3. How long has he or she been an administrator?

4. Where did he or she get training and experience?

5. Ask to see the home's license. What is the date of the last inspection?

NOTE: If the administrator won't let you see the license or if the home doesn't have a license, *LEAVE NOW!*

6. Ask to see the results of the latest state inspection. Are they good?

Yes_____ No_____

7. Is the home a Medicare/Medicaid-certified facility?

Yes_____ No_____

NOTE: If it isn't, *LEAVE NOW!*

8. Are ALL residents' rooms certified for Medicare/Medicaid?

Yes_____ No_____

9. Does the home accept residents already on Medicaid?

Yes_____ No_____

10. Does the home give preference to residents on Medicare?

Yes_____ No_____

11. If so, what does the home do when a resident's Medicare coverage runs out?

12. What is the home's bed hold policy?

13. Does the home have a special unit for residents with Alzheimer's disease or other types of dementia?

Yes_____ No_____

14. If so, does that special unit have trained staff to care for those residents?

Yes_____ No_____

15. What activities does the home provide for the residents in the special unit?

16. What are the names of the staff doctors?

17. How often does each doctor visit the home?

18. Is the doctor's name and telephone number given to the resident and the family?

Yes_____ No_____

19. Who takes care of the residents when the doctor isn't available?

20. Are relatives notified immediately when there's a change in the resident's condition?

Yes_____ No_____

21. Does the home allow a resident to choose his or her own physician even if that physician is NOT on the staff?

Yes_____ No_____

22. Is the Director of Nursing Services a Registered Nurse?

Yes_____ No_____

23. Is at least one Registered Nurse or LPN on duty at ALL times, night and day, seven days a week?

Yes_____ No_____

24. What is the ratio of nurses to residents? _____

25. Does the home use temporary staff hired from outside the home?

Yes_____ No_____

26. Does the home provide physical, occupational, and speech therapies?

Yes_____ No_____

27. Who provides them?

28. How often and how long are they given?

29. What arrangements does the home have for dental, hearing, and vision care?

30. Does the home have a full-time social service director?

Yes_____ No_____

31. Does the home have a full-time activity director?

Yes_____ No_____

32. Is there a list of any rules residents must follow?

Yes_____ No_____

33. If so, ask to see it. Do you think the rules are reasonable?

Yes_____ No_____

34. Does the home have a Resident Council?

Yes_____ No_____

35. What are some recent suggestions from the Resident Council?

36. Are family members allowed to attend the Resident Council meetings?

Yes_____ No_____

37. Is there a Family Council as well?

Yes_____ No_____

38. Are there any restrictions on visiting hours at any time, day or evening?

Yes_____ No_____

39. What are the requirements of the local law or fire code for emergencies?

40. How is the staff trained for emergencies like fire and how often is training held?

41. How many fire drills does the home have each year?

42. Is there a working sprinkler system as well as fire extinguishers?

Yes_____ No_____

43. Are there any extra charges that aren't included in the basic daily rate?

Yes_____ No_____

44. If so, will the administrator give you a list of all extra charges?

Yes_____ No_____

45. Does the home handle residents' money if given written authorization?

Yes_____ No_____

46. How does the home handle that money?

47. Do residents get quarterly reports on their finances?

Yes_____ No_____

48. Is there a personal banking system set up in the home for residents to use, especially for spending money?

Yes_____ No_____

49. Does the home provide beauty and barber services?

Yes_____ No_____

50. Do residents have a telephone in their rooms or close by?

Yes_____ No_____

51. Are there any restrictions on residents making or receiving telephone calls?

Yes_____ No_____

52. Are residents allowed to have their own radio and television in their rooms?

Yes_____ No_____

53. Are they allowed to bring some favorite furniture, like a chair and chest of drawers, from home?

Yes_____ No_____

54. Will the administrator give you a copy of the admissions contract?

Yes_____ No_____

55. Will the administrator sign YOUR copy of this questionnaire in which you've written his or her answers?

Yes_____ No_____

56. If not, will he or she read the extra copy and fill in the blanks and *sign it*?

Yes_____ No_____

57. Will the administrator take you on a personal tour of the home?

Yes_____ No_____

Letter to the Administrator

Dear Administrator,

I am sorry that I was not able to meet with you at this time. I am very interested in your facility and would like to know more about it. To that end, I have interviewed a staff member from your administration office. I also have asked your office to deliver this letter to you along with a copy of the questions I asked your staff member. I would appreciate it very much if you would take the time to write down your answers so that I will have my information directly from you. I would also greatly appreciate it if you would sign your copy.

Thank you very much for taking the time to fill out this questionnaire. I look forward to receiving your answers as soon as possible since I am working within a short time frame to find the right facility and must make my decision very soon.

Yours Truly,

_____

(Signature)

Checklist for Nursing Home Staff Doctors

This is a quick check of the home's staff doctors and can be done any time after your interview on Day 3. You got their names from the administrator or admissions coordinator. Now you're going to call the local hospitals to check the credentials of the home's doctors. Hospitals have this information on file and it's open to the public.

Start your telephone call by identifying yourself and saying that you're looking at nursing homes for a loved one. Mention the name of the nursing home you're interested in. Tell the person on the other end of the line that you would like some information about the home's staff doctors. You'll be connected to someone who can answer your questions. Keep this list beside you when you make the calls, and ask the following questions about EACH doctor on your list:

1. Is Doctor _____ on staff at this hospital?

   Yes_____ No_____

2. If not, is he or she affiliated with this hospital?

   Yes_____ No_____

3. How long has Dr. _____ been on your staff or affiliated with your hospital?

4. What is this doctor's specialty?

5. Where did Dr. _____ get his/her medical training?

6. Where did Dr. _____ receive his/her degree in Medicine from?

Chapter 4

DAY 4: INTERVIEWING OTHER STAFF MEMBERS

This is going to be a busy day for you if you were able to line up interviews with the social service director, the activity director, and the dietitian. The interviews won't take long, although inspecting activity resources might add a bit more time to your visit. However, the time spent on these interviews is very important to your investigation. So, let's begin by giving you a run-down on the three positions and what to look for.

THE SOCIAL SERVICE DIRECTOR

As I mentioned earlier, if the home has more than 120 beds, it must employ a full-time social service director. Homes that are smaller often have a social service director on a consultant basis.

The role of the social service director is very important to a new resident's adjustment to the home. Moving to a nursing home is a major change in a person's life; one that requires help in dealing with loneliness, fear, grief, depression, and anxiety. The skills of a well-trained social service director will help your loved one adjust as smoothly as possible to this new life.

The ideal social service director is one who's working in the home because he or she loves the elderly. Unfortunately, some social workers take jobs in nursing homes while waiting for a better job opportunity. Generally speaking, these are the ones who don't measure up to the standards you want.

You'll find the checklist for this interview at the end of this chapter. The questions are presented here with extra comments and tips.

1. What are the social service director's qualifications?

You want to find out what kind of degree he or she has and from where.

2. What are his or her responsibilities?

Write down the responses. They should include:

- helping individual residents cope with the stress of loneliness, grief, depression and anxiety about moving into the home;
- holding workshops or counseling groups for staff and for residents' family members;
- being familiar with the family history and health of each resident so that he or she can be consulted if a resident's family has any questions or problems about the care or daily life of their loved one;
- being familiar with all services that are provided to the residents and their families by the various social services available in the community;
- working with the rest of the staff on common problems arising with residents' interaction with each other or with the staff.

3. In what specific ways does the social service director help new residents adjust?

Moving to a nursing home is a traumatic event in a person's life, no matter how good the place is. A well-trained social service director can play a major role in helping the new resident adjust positively to the new environment. He or she can educate the staff, as well as the relatives, about any problems a new resident might have adjusting to the home.

4. Is the social service director also acting as activity director for the home?

If planning and monitoring activities is part of the job, my advice is to forget the place.

5. Ask the social service director to take you on a tour of the home.

Observe the reactions between the social service director and the residents. Look for genuine interest and even affection being expressed. Residents know who loves them and who doesn't. I've seen residents who can't speak, hear, or see throw out their arms for a hug when they sense the presence of a truly caring social service director. That's the sort of thing you want to see.

6. When you take the tour of the home with the social service director, watch to see if he or she pays more attention to the staff than to the residents.

You want a social service director who treats the residents (not the staff) as the most important people in the home.

THE ACTIVITY DIRECTOR

It's important that you also check to see if the home has a trained activity director. Often, there is no one really qualified to oversee activities.

Many small nursing homes leave this area up to the overworked staff. Feeble attempts are made by workers who don't have the time or the talent to keep the residents happily occupied. This often leads to endless hours of bingo or children's card games or simply watching TV. It's a terrible thing to see intelligent residents desperately trying to keep mentally alert when there's nothing to do. A well-trained, people-oriented activity director is worth his or her weight in gold. If you're told the facility doesn't have one, cross the place off your list!

You'll find the checklist for this interview at the end of this chapter.

1. What activities does the home provide?

Ask the activity director to describe each one and take notes about them as they are described. Activities should include:

- physical therapy
- music therapy
- gardening
- library books, audio books
- birthday parties
- church services on the premises
- volunteer groups
- lectures
- shopping outings
- pet therapy
- arts and crafts
- woodworking
- painting
- card games
- movies

■ sing-a-longs

With a capable activity director on the staff, the list can be endless.

2. What activities are there for residents who are bedridden or who aren't interested in group activities?

State policy requires that there must be planned activities for all residents, including those who are bedridden. Too many homes don't provide any form of activity for those residents who can't get out of their rooms. This is unacceptable. One of the worst cases I saw was in a home where the staff had hung a baby's crib mobile over the head of a bedridden resident. This was considered an activity! A good activity director will provide regular volunteer visitations, pet therapy, audio cassettes of books, touch therapy, and music therapy, just to name a few. There is no excuse for letting a bedridden or room-bound resident be shut out of activities.

3. Ask the activity director to give you a guided tour of the home.

Watch the reactions between residents and the activity director. Is he or she warm and friendly? Do the residents seem happy to see him or her?

4. Ask to see the activity resources.

There should be lots of books with large print, cassette tapes, and tape players. Check the tape players to see if they're in working condition. You want to see for yourself! I've been in nursing homes where there were just two or three cassette players and none of them had batteries. If a home has a sewing room or a kiln, check to see if it's being used. These special features look great, but many homes don't have the staff or time to oversee their use. Consequently, the residents never get a chance to enjoy them.

5. Talk to the residents about the activities.

Ask them what their favorite ones are and if they think there are enough things to do in the home.

6. Check out the activity board.

Look for an activity board in the main dining room and on all floors. This board should be in large print. It should display all scheduled activities for the week or month. Unfortunately, in many homes the activity board looks great, but the activities don't exist. Why? Most states, by law, require regular activities to be *planned*, and the schedule must be very *visible*. Friends and relatives assume that all those scheduled activities are actually happening. They read the board and say, "Oh look, Dad, you're going to love it here! They've got woodworking and bridge and bingo and movies and lectures. Oh, this is wonderful!" Many times, the staff is too small and overworked to carry out the plans. Your dad could end up watching television from breakfast until bedtime. Check it out. Not just once, but several times. *What looks good on the board may not ever happen in that home.*

7. Copy down the activities from the board.

You'll need to refer to them later when you make another visit to the home. You want to see if the activities that are scheduled actually happen. On your next visit, check to see if the activity scheduled on the board is in progress. Have your friends check this schedule out during their visits as well.

THE DIETITIAN

One of the greatest sources of pleasure for the residents is mealtime. Check out the food and its preparation. Ask yourself if you'd enjoy eating in that "restaurant" every day for the rest of *your* life.

Every nursing home should have a professionally trained dietitian since many residents have special nutritional needs. The dietitian should be willing to consult with you about special dietary needs *and* to provide them whenever possible.

The checklist for this interview is at the end of this chapter.

1. How long has the dietitian been at that home?

This question will give you an idea of how familiar he or she is with the residents' individual dietary needs.

2. What are his or her qualifications?

He or she doesn't have to be a gourmet chef, but you want someone who has training in special dietary needs of the elderly and who's had plenty of cooking experience.

3. How will he or she attend to the dietary needs of your loved one?

List those needs and ask how the dietitian would handle them.

4. Ask the dietitian if the administrator and staff eat the same food as the residents.

Unfortunately, in many homes the food is so unappetizing that the staff won't eat it. Watch the dietitian's facial expression when you ask this question. Does he or she laugh or look angry or uncomfortable? These could be signs that something is wrong. If the staff won't eat the food, why should the residents?

5. Notice the dietitian's attitude towards your questioning.

Is he or she genuinely friendly? Does he or she seem to take a real interest in your questions?

6. Is the dietitian neat in appearance?

Is he or she wearing a clean uniform or apron? I've seen dietitians with grubby uniforms and two days' worth of grime on their aprons! This doesn't say much for the cleanliness of the kitchen or the quality of the food.

7. Take a tour of the kitchen.

Any home that refuses your request to inspect the kitchen should be crossed off your list! You should be allowed to take the tour when *you* want to, *not* when the staff can arrange it. I feel strongly about this because I once saw cockroaches baked in the cornbread! So take the tour on your terms or forget the place.

8. Check out the weekly or monthly menu.

Is it well balanced, or does it include fried foods, too much starch and not enough fruits and vegetables? And is it a varied menu? The same food day after day gets monotonous quickly.

9. Order the main meal of the day and taste it.

Visitors should always be welcomed to buy a meal. Don't feel embarrassed to ask. Check to see how it's cooked. Is it fried? Are the vegetables tasty or have they been steamed until they have no color, taste, or nutrients? Is the food served attractively, or does it at least look edible? Is the food served at appropriate temperatures? Is it served on time?

10. Check the quantity of the food.

Is there plenty of food on the dinner plates? Take a good look at the residents. Do they look as though they're getting enough to eat, or are many of them noticeably underweight?

11. Check the posted menu.

Then check to see if the meal on the menu is actually being served that day. Check this on each visit. Some nursing homes post great menus but don't really serve them to the residents.

12. If you're visiting during a meal time, check what's going on in the dining room.

Are the residents eating well and receiving assistance if needed? Is the staff big enough to help feed those who can't feed themselves? It's difficult to open a milk carton or cut a piece of meat when your hands are crippled by arthritis or a stroke. Many times I've fed residents when the people hired to do the job were nowhere around. I've seen elderly people crying because no one was there to help them eat the food in front of them.

13. Check the rooms of bedridden residents at the same meal time.

Are they being served? Are they getting help from staff or do they have to wait for assistance while their food gets cold? Go back and check them again in twenty minutes. Are they still waiting?

CHECKLISTS FOR DAY 4

Questions for the Social Service Director

Use this checklist either on a clipboard or directly from the book. Don't feel uncomfortable about asking these questions, the social service director expects them.

1. What kind of degree does the social service director have?

2. Where is the degree from?

3. What are the social service director's responsibilities?

4. How do the social service director and the rest of the staff help the new residents adjust to the home?

5. Does the social service director also act as the activity director?

Yes_____ No_____

6. Ask the social service director to take you on a tour of the home. Make the following observations during the tour:

a) Watch the reaction between the residents and the social service director. Is there genuine interest or affection expressed? Yes_____ No_____

b) Does the social service director pay more attention to the staff than to the residents? Yes_____ No_____

Questions for the Activity Director

The following checklist should be used the same way as the checklist for the social service director. Simply ask the questions straight out of the book or from a clipboard. Again, remember that the activity director will expect these sorts of questions.

1. What activities does the home provide?

2. What activities are provided for bedridden residents?

3. What activities are provided for residents who aren't interested in group activities?

4. Ask the activity director to take you on a personal tour. Are the reactions between the residents and the activity director warm and friendly?

   Yes_____ No_____

5. Ask to see the activity resources. The following should be some of the resources you find:

   Books (lots!) Yes_____ No_____

   Large print books Yes_____ No_____

   Audio cassettes of books and the Bible Yes_____ No_____

   Tape players that work Yes_____ No_____

Other resources?

6. Talk to residents about the activities. Do they think there are enough activities in the home?

Yes_____ No_____

7. Is there an activity board in the dining room?

Yes_____ No_____

8. Is there an activity board on all floors or wings of the home?

Yes_____ No_____

9. Are the activities listed in large print?

Yes_____ No_____

10. Copy down the activities from the board.

Be sure to check to see if these activities are really happening. You can do this on your next visit which can be scheduled at the same time as one or two of the activities.

11. Be sure to give copies of the activity board list to your helpers who will be visiting at different times of the day.

By comparing notes, you'll be able to see if the activities on the board are actually held. This is *very* important!

Questions for the Dietitian

This is an important part of your investigation because you want to make sure the meals your loved one will be eating are well-balanced, plentiful, tasty, served on time, served at the proper temperatures, and prepared in a clean kitchen.

1. How long has the dietitian been at the home?

2. How is he or she qualified?

    Training

    Experience

3. Tell the dietitian any nutritional needs your loved one has. How will he or she attend to those needs?

4. Do the administrator and the staff eat the same meals as the residents?

    Yes_____ No_____

5. What is the dietitian's attitude towards your questions?

    Friendly and helpful _____
    Not friendly or helpful _____

6. Is the dietitian wearing a clean apron or uniform?

    Yes_____ No_____

7. Did you take a tour of the kitchen?

    Yes_____ No_____

8. Is the kitchen clean (appliances, counter tops, floor, ceiling fans, walls, etc.)?

Yes_____ No_____

9. Is food properly refrigerated?

Yes_____ No_____

10. Is the weekly or monthly menu well-balanced and varied?

Yes_____ No_____

11. Were you able to buy or sample a meal and, if so, was it tasty, well-prepared, and balanced?

Yes_____ No_____

12. Check the size of the servings. Are they plentiful?

Yes_____ No_____

13. Is the meal that's being served the meal that is actually listed on the menu for the day?

Yes_____ No_____

14. Is assistance being given to residents who need help eating?

Yes_____ No_____

15. Are the bedridden residents being served at the same time as the other residents?

Yes_____ No_____

16. Are the bedridden residents receiving help to eat?

Yes_____ No_____

17. If not, did they receive help within 20 minutes?

Yes_____ No_____

Chapter 5

DAY 5: SATURDAY AFTERNOON INSPECTION

SURPRISE INSPECTION

To do a complete investigation, you absolutely *must* make one more visit to the home, and it *must* be on Saturday! Since staffs are usually smaller on weekends, any problems that do exist will be quite visible. The best time to go is around a meal time, preferably about 4:30 or 5:00 p.m. Observing a meal time when staff is smaller can be a real eye-opener to the overall treatment of residents.

Another reason for this Saturday visit is to check out the safety features and to get another look at the environment of the home. This is easier to do when the staff is smaller. You'll have fewer distractions and you'll have a chance to catch those few details you didn't see during your other visits.

The checklists for these inspections are at the end of this chapter. It won't take long, but if you don't do this surprise check, you'll never really know for sure what goes on behind those nursing home doors when you're not there. So grit your teeth and go back there one more time.

1. Check out the restraints on residents.

Do you see more residents in restraints than you did during the week? This can happen when the staff is smaller, but it really should not occur.

2. Are residents sitting in their own excrement or urine?

This is another infraction that happens when there is a smaller staff.

3. Do you think the smaller staff can handle the workload?

Some nursing homes cut the weekend staff so far back that it's impossible to care for all the residents properly.

4. Is there a registered nurse (RN) or licensed practical nurse (LPN) on duty?

There is no excuse for one not being on duty at all times during the weekend as well as throughout the week.

5. Are call buttons being answered within a reasonable time?

Note flashing call lights at the beginning and end of your visit. Are they the same ones?

6. Do you hear residents calling for help?

This is another sign that the staff is too small or not attentive. This is a common occurrence on Saturdays.

7. Walk through the area where the bedridden residents live.

Are they getting attention? Are they clean or are they lying in their own excrement or calling for help? Again, this happens often on Saturdays without the proper staff.

8. Are there any activities scheduled and, if so, are they occurring?

Check the activity board or your notes and then check to see if scheduled activities are really happening.

9. If a meal is being served, are residents who need help being assisted by aides?

Or are they just sitting in front of their food, unable to feed themselves? Are there enough aides to help? As I mentioned earlier, I've seen residents crying because no one was there to help them. Those who suffer from strokes or arthritis, for example, often can't use a knife, fork, or spoon or even open a carton of milk without some help.

10. Are the bedridden residents being served at the same time as the other residents?

In some homes they have to wait until all others are served since the staff is smaller. They end up being very hungry and eating cold, unappetizing meals.

11. Are the bedridden residents being helped to eat?

Again, smaller staff means the weaker residents sometimes wait the longest. Sometimes the food is just brought in, left for a while and then removed. Check it out.

12. Are the residents being served the meal that is posted on the menu for that Saturday?

Sometimes the menu is changed at the last minute and residents are not served a good, complete meal.

13. Do you see aides grouped together talking instead of attending to residents?

This also occurs more often on weekends.

CHECKING SAFETY AND THE ENVIRONMENT

Keeping in mind that the facility will be your loved one's home will help you focus on details that can affect quality of life in the home. It doesn't have to be fancy, but it must be clean, safe, and comfortable. It's very important that you do your own checking on safety features and the comfort level of the home. Bear in mind that your loved one would be living 24 hours a day with any problems you find! To get a good picture of the safety and comfort provided, use the checklist.

- Are there handrails in all corridors?
- Do you see a sprinkler system and the number of fire extinguishers required by the local fire code?

- Are the exit doors supervised or do they have safety alarms so that people can't wander in and out?

- Can wheelchairs get through all doors and halls, including fire exits?

- Are there grab bars, safety mats, and call lights in the bathrooms, and do the call lights work?

- Are there call lights in the bedrooms and do they work?

- Are the residents' rooms clean and attractive?

- How many people share a room? Is there enough space?

- Is the home warm (or cool) enough?

- Does the home have air-conditioning?

- Do you see any residents sitting directly under the air conditioning vents? This happens in some homes and the cold can aggravate residents' aches and pains.

- Are there bathrooms in each room? How many residents have to share a bathroom?

- Is it too bright or too dark in the halls, rooms and dining room?

- Is the volume of the PA system comfortable, or is it too loud or too soft?

CHECKLISTS FOR DAY 5

Surprise Inspection

This Saturday inspection will help you *really* see what goes on when the staff is smaller. It's very important that you go during mealtime, preferably about 4:30 to 5 in the afternoon. Take special note of the following:

1. Are there more residents in restraints than there were during your other visits?

    Yes_____ No_____

2. Are residents sitting in their own excrement or urine?

    Yes_____ No_____

3. Is there enough staff to handle the workload?

    Yes_____ No_____

4. Is there a registered nurse (RN) or licensed practical nurse (LPN) on duty?

    Yes_____ No_____

5. Are call buttons being answered promptly?

    Yes_____ No_____

6. Do you hear residents calling for help?

    Yes_____ No_____

7. Are the bedridden residents receiving the amount of attention they need?

    Yes_____ No_____

8. Are there any activities going on for the residents?

Yes_____ No_____

9. Are the activities that are scheduled actually taking place?

Yes_____ No_____

10. If your visit is during mealtime, are those who need assistance being helped by the aides?

Yes_____ No_____

11. Are the bedridden residents being served their meal at the same time as the other residents?

Yes_____ No_____

12. Are the bedridden residents being helped to eat their food?

Yes_____ No_____

13. Is the meal that's posted on the menu the same as the meal actually being served?

Yes_____ No_____

14. Do you see aides talking in small groups instead of attending to the residents' needs?

Yes_____ No_____

15. Now do your Safety and Environment Check (see next checklist).

Safety Features and the Environment

This check won't take long and will give you a good idea of how safe and comfortable the home is.

1. Are there handrails in all corridors?

Yes_____ No_____

2. Is there a sprinkler system?

Yes_____ No_____

3. Are there enough fire extinguishers?

Yes_____ No_____

4. Are the exit doors supervised or do they have safety alarms?

Yes_____ No_____

5. Are all doors, halls, and fire exits wide enough for wheelchairs to get through?

Yes_____ No_____

6. Check bathrooms for:

grab bars Yes_____ No_____

safety mats Yes_____ No_____

call buttons Yes_____ No_____

7. Are there call lights or buttons in the bedrooms?

Yes_____ No_____

8. Do the call lights in the bathrooms and bedrooms work?

Yes_____ No_____

9. Are they within easy reach for residents in wheelchairs or beds?

Yes_____ No_____

10. Are the residents' rooms clean and attractive?

Yes_____ No_____

11. How many people share a room?_____

12. Is there enough space for each resident in the shared rooms?

Yes_____ No_____

13. Is the home warm enough or cool enough for the season?

Yes_____ No_____

14. Does the home have air-conditioning?

Yes_____ No_____

15. Are there bathrooms in each room?

Yes_____ No_____

16. If not, how many residents must share a bathroom?_____

17. Is the lighting in the rooms, halls and dining room at a comfortable level (not too bright or too dark)?

Yes_____ No_____

18. Is the volume of the PA system comfortable?

Yes_____ No_____

Chapter 6

SOME FINAL THOUGHTS

By following this 5-day plan, you'll get a clear overall picture of the nursing home. It involves hard work, but it's designed to be completed in just one week, if necessary, assuming that your interviews can be arranged within that time. By using the checklists, tips and information provided throughout the book, you'll find the guidance you need to do a complete, panic-free investigation. *And don't let administrators, nursing staff, or any other personnel intimidate you!* Ask all the questions and insist on getting answers. Keep your eyes open. Know your rights as a consumer. Be aggressive and thorough in your investigation. Remember, you're the buyer; the administrator and staff want to sell.

Finding a good care facility is a challenge. But, by using this guide and getting your helpers involved as much as possible, you *will* find the right place. And the rewards will be immeasurable because, when the work is done and you've made your decision, your loved one will receive the care he or she deserves, and you'll have peace of mind knowing you did everything you could to find the best nursing home possible!

In closing, let me share the following two situations I experienced during my 20 years working in nursing homes. My wish is that all nursing homes were like the one in the second story. The reality is that there are too many like the one in the first. Many fall somewhere in between.

I also wish you the very best in your search for an excellent home for your loved one. To that end, I dedicate this book with the knowledge that it will guide you in the right direction and arm you with enough information to help you see beyond the surface of any nursing home into the very *heart* of the place, for that is what your search is really all about.

JESSIE

This true story happened in a facility in a southern state where I was a volunteer. One morning as I was helping a resident write a letter, I heard a shout. "Missy! Come quick! Jessie's fallen!"

I ran into the hall and found Jessie crumpled on the floor, her hand clutching a white cane. "Jessie! Jessie! Can you hear me?" I asked as I cradled her head in my lap.

"Yes'm, I hears you," Jessie whispered.

"What happened, Jessie? Are you all right?" Jessie didn't answer. Her eyes stared blindly at the ceiling.

"Luther, did you see what happened?" I asked the old man who had shouted for help.

"Yes'm, I see. Jessie, she just walkin' down the hall one minute and the next thing I know she just went down. Nobody near her. She don't trip. Just went down like a rock."

"Jessie, do you hurt anywhere?"

"My head feels...funny and...legs...won't work," Jessie mumbled.

I grasped Jessie's wrist and found her pulse faint and irregular. "Luther, please get the orderly and tell him to bring a wheelchair. And get the nurse," I said. Luther hobbled quickly down the hall while I tended to Jessie. As I bent over her, whispers and shuffling feet surrounded us.

Looking up, I gazed into a circle of frightened faces. The residents huddled together, nodding their heads and sneaking glances over their shoulders.

"Missy, is she all right?"

"Missy, you watch out!"

"Missy, you be careful. Nurse Becker, she be mad."

Nurse Becker was the head nurse during the day and the residents were afraid of her. She was rigid, cold. She was cruel in subtle ways, like denying a resident a favorite dessert if he or she had been incontinent in the dining room or had spilled coffee on the floor. She often screamed at residents when they moved slowly or defied her in any way. But she was a close friend of the administrator and the two of them would not tolerate any complaints from the staff or residents.

Within minutes, the orderly hurried towards us, pushing a wheelchair and looking behind him. "She's comin' this way, Missy. You in big trouble now," he muttered as he helped me get Jessie into the wheelchair.

"What do you think you're doing?" Nurse Becker screamed as she marched towards us. "Who gave you permission to get that wheelchair?" she demanded, shoving residents out of her way.

"Something's wrong with Jessie," I stated. "She just collapsed. She says her head feels funny and her legs are weak."

Nurse Becker grasped the arms of the wheelchair and crouched down face-to-face with Jessie. "Now you listen to me, Jessie," she ordered. "You know you're just puttin' on an act. Get out of this chair right now! You don't fool me one bit. Come on, get up and get your butt back to your room!"

The residents gasped and backed away. "Jessie's not pretending," I said. "She really can't walk. I think she may have had a stroke."

"And just who do you think you are, a nurse?" Nurse Becker snapped back. "Get out of my way while I tend to Jessie. Jessie, you get up right now and get walkin!" And, grabbing her under the arms, Nurse Becker hauled Jessie to her feet. With a kick, she sent the wheelchair reeling down the hall. "Luther, give Jessie her cane!" she ordered. "There. Now walk, Jessie! You hear me? Walk!"

Jessie slowly straightened until she stood her full height, six feet tall and regal. Head held high, she began to walk, dazed and unsteady, back to her room. The thump, thump, thump of her cane tolled through the silent hall. I ran after her as Nurse Becker screamed at me to keep away. Jessie refused my help and just kept walking. I'll never forget her proud old back as she made her way down that hall.

The staff found Jessie dead the next morning. The doctor said it was a stroke. Nurse Becker said it was just her time to go.

GEORGE

I remember the first time I walked into the special care unit of one large nursing home. The unit was for residents suffering from Alzheimer's disease. I was working as a music therapist at the time and had come for my first visit to direct a sing-along for the residents.

When I stepped off the elevator, I was stunned. Perched on the nurse's desk was a bright green parakeet in a big red cage. He was chatting quietly to a tiny lady who stood smiling right next to him. Along the walls hung multi-colored tapestries, hooked rugs, and macramé weavings. Laughter floated down the hall and someone was whistling. Suddenly, a young, heavyset woman and a thin, old man twirled around the corner in a gentle waltz. She wore a pink smock and he was humming *Daisy, Daisy, give me your answer do!* She was an aide on the staff and he was one of the residents. They almost bumped into me as he spun her around for one last time. Both of them burst out laughing. "Thanks, George," she said, grinning up at him. He didn't answer her. His eyes were on my guitar case.

"I bet that's a violin in there," he said. "I used to fiddle a bit." And George began a steady stream of verbal memories. Yes, they were muddled, the years mixed up, names and sentences coming fast and in no particular order. But George was excited and eager to reminisce.

We stood there listening for a few minutes and then the aide put her arm around him and said, "George, I love your stories and I don't want to interrupt. But let's help the music lady get ready for a sing-along, okay?"

George bent down, grabbed my guitar case and began walking back down the hall to the dining room. "Well, come on!" he shouted over his shoulder.

The aide laughed and called, "We'll be right there!" She turned to me and said, "Hi, I'm Carol and you just met George. He's having a good day today. He's been here since his wife died three years ago and half the time he's still grieving for her. Music perks him up but don't be surprised if he cries too."

As we walked towards the dining room, Carol told me a bit about the other residents. There were fifteen in the unit, all at different stages of

Alzheimer's disease and all very special in her eyes. She called them "The Family."

Just before we entered the dining room, I told her I'd never seen such beautiful tapestries on any other nursing home walls. "Oh, aren't they great?" she replied. "The Family loves them. You know, some of them are in advanced stages of Alzheimer's and they can't communicate anymore. But they love those wall hangings. Just watch and you'll see them running their hands all over them." She was right. After that first day, whenever I visited the unit I noticed two or three residents touching those tapestries, twisting the fabrics between their fingers and studying the bright colors.

The dining room was small with just enough tables and chairs for The Family. One entire wall consisted of windows looking onto a green meadow that stretched the imagination. Cows grazed under willow trees and an old log fence zigzagged towards the horizon. "Wow! What a view!" I whispered.

"Give me a few minutes to get The Family together before you start," Carol said, and she left me standing in a trance by that window.

"Hey, are you going to play or what?"

I turned around to see George sitting in the corner with my guitar case. "I sure am, George," I said. "My name's Missy and I'd love to have you help me."

"You bet!" he declared as he started to open the case. "Well, I'll be darned if that's not the best fiddle I ever saw!" he said as he lifted my guitar into the air the way a priest lifts up a chalice. "We're in for a pretty good time." His eyes shone into mine and we became good friends right then.

He didn't remember me from one visit to the next, but I'll never forget dear George. And he put me through my paces and kept me on my toes! "Hey, can you play *Take Me Out to the Ball Game*?" "Hey, can you play *My Wild Irish Rose*?" His requests were endless. And many times I would catch him crying. He would say to The Family, "You'll have to excuse me but my wife died yesterday and this was our favorite song."

Every time George became upset, the nurse or an aide would be right there. "Come on, George, dance with me." "Hey, George! Got a minute?

Give me a spin around the room!" And off he'd go waltzing through tangos and marches and hymns, comforted and content.

The best thing about the staff was that they treated each member of The Family the same way. No matter when I went, with my guitar or without, I always found the same atmosphere. I tried every tip I've told you in this book to catch that staff at a disadvantage. I always found them consistently loving and warm to every resident, night or day.

As for George? He still doesn't know me from one visit to the next, but he's still dancing.

Appendix A

RESIDENT'S RIGHTS

1. Free Choice.

You have the following rights regarding your medical treatment in a nursing home:

- The right to choose a doctor. The doctor must comply with certain federal regulations regarding your care or the home may replace your doctor after notifying you.
- Full information given to you in advance about changes in your care or treatment that affect your well-being. This includes full information on your total health situation. It also includes your right to refuse treatment.
- The right to choose someone to act as your agent when and if you are no longer able to make your own decisions about your health care.
- The right to agree to participate in experimental research.

2. Freedom from Abuse and Restraints.

You will be free from any abuse or punishment including physical, sexual, or mental abuse, corporal punishment, and involuntary seclusion. Chemical and physical restraints will only be used if they are needed to treat your medical problem and then only to ensure your safety or the safety of other residents. You or your legal representative or family members will be consulted before restraints are used unless in an emergency situation.

3. <u>Privacy</u>.

You are entitled to privacy in your accommodations. This also includes the right to privacy during medical treatment and during personal hygiene care. You also have the right to receive and send mail unopened and to make telephone calls. You have the right to receive visitors.

4. <u>Confidentiality</u>.

You have the right to inspect your records. Your medical, social, and financial records will be released only to the members of the staff who need them, to another care facility if you have to be moved, or when required by law or the agency that pays for your care.

5. <u>Accommodation of Needs</u>.

You have the right to make choices regarding any needs that specifically affect your life (for example, individual dietary needs or preferences).

6. <u>Voice Grievances</u>.

You have the right to voice grievances to the nursing home without fear of reprisal.

7. <u>Resident Group</u>.

You have the right to organize a resident council or to participate in one. Any written recommendations from the council pertaining to policy and decisions that affect life and care in the home must be considered by the staff at the home.

8. <u>Participation in Activities</u>.

You have the right to participate in any activity that does not infringe on other residents' rights. You also have the right to participate in any of the home's scheduled activities that you find interesting. You have all rights of citizenship including the right to vote. You also have the right to worship as you choose.

9. <u>The Facility's License</u>.

You have the right to read the home's latest state inspection report, including plans to correct any deficiencies found.

10. <u>Funds</u>.

You have the right to manage your own money. You also have the right to have the home manage your funds in an interest-bearing account upon your request. You have the right to receive quarterly statements.

11. <u>Complaints to the State</u>.

You have the right to report any abuse or neglect you think you have experienced in the home to the state. You have the right to file a complaint if any of your property has been stolen.

12. <u>Advocacy Groups</u>.

You have the right to be given information about advocacy groups and the ombudsman in your area.

13. <u>Visitors</u>.

You have the right to receive an unlimited number of visits with family, the ombudsman, your doctor, and government agency representatives. You also have the right to refuse to visit with any of these people.

14. <u>Personal Possessions</u>.

You have the right to a comfortable, homelike environment and to use your personal belongings in such a way that will not hinder health and safety regulations.

15. <u>Notification of Change</u>.

You have the right to be notified (along with your doctor, a family member, and your legal representative) of any change in your condition or significant change in treatment. This notification must be within 24 hours of the change.

16. <u>Bed Hold Policy</u>.

If your care is being paid by Medicaid, the state will pay to hold your bed for 15 days if you need to be hospitalized. It can be extended to a total of 20 days if ordered by your doctor. If you pay for your own care, you must pay the full daily rate for each day that your bed is held.

Appendix B

OTHER RESOURCES AND PUBLICATIONS

ORGANIZATIONS

Health Care Financing Administration
7500 Security Blvd.
Baltimore, MD 21244-1850
http://www.hcfa.gov

Alzheimer's Association
70 E. Lake Street
Suite 600
Chicago, IL 60601
(312) 853-3060

American Association of Retired Persons
601 E Street, N.W.
Washington, DC 20049

Canadian Association of Retired Persons
27 Queen St. East, Suite 1304
Toronto, Ontario M5C 2M6 CANADA

For information about Medicare contact the
Social Security Administration
1 (800) 772-1213

For information about your state's nursing homes, contact
Citizens for Better Care
1 (800) 292-7852

For general information in Canada, contact
Ministry of Health (Ottawa)
(613) 957-2991 or (613) 954-8616

BOOKS

The Medicare & Medicaid Guide to Choosing a Nursing Home
(Publication No.HCFA 02174)
U.S. Department of Health and Human Services
Health Care Financing Administration
7500 Security Blvd.
Baltimore, MD 21244-1850

The Inside Guide to America's Nursing Homes: Rankings & Ratings for Every Nursing Home in the U.S., 1998-1999
by Robert N. Bua
Published by Warner Books (ISBN 0446673080)

The Baby Boomer's Guide to Caring for Aging Parents
by Bart Astor
Published by McMillan General Reference (ISBN 0028616170)

Beat the Nursing Home Trap: A Consumer's Guide to Choosing & Financing Long-Term Care
by Joseph L. Matthews
Published by Nolo Press (ISBN 0873372301)

The Human Factor in Nursing Home Care
by David B. Oliver & Sally Tureman
Published by Haworth Press (ISBN 0866567321)

Life Worth Living: How Someone You Love Can Still Enjoy Life in a Nursing Home
by William H. Thomas
Published by Vanderwyk and Burnham (ISBN 0964108968)

The Medicaid Planning Handbook: A Guide to Protecting Your Family's Assets from Catastrophic Nursing Home Costs (2nd Rev. Ed.)
by Alexander A. Bove, Jr.
Published by Little, Brown and Co., Inc. (ISBN 0316103748)

Nursing Homes: Getting Good Care There
by Sarah Greene Burger, Virginia Fraser, Sara Hunt & Barbara Frank
Published by Impact Christian Books (ISBN 0915166976)

Enhancing the Self-Esteem of the Nursing Home Resident
by Marylou Hughes
Published by M & H Publishing Co. (ISBN 1877735167)

How to Achieve Quality of Life & Care in a Nursing Home
by Elizabeth Yeh & Edward Rosenwasser
Published by Rosewater Publishing Co. (ISBN 0932495109)

INDEX

Social Security, 7
   Social Security Administration, 8
social service director, 21-22, 35, 49-51
staff, 2-4, 6, 10, 13-20, 22-23, 29, 31-35, 37, 50-58, 65-68, 75, 82-83
state inspection report, 14, 30-31, 83

T

temporary nursing care, 3
therapy, 34, 37, 52-53

V

volunteer, 1-2

W

waiting list, 1-3
wheelchairs, 15, 20-21, 69

ABOUT THE AUTHOR

Born and raised in Ontario, Canada, Ms. Kraatz married an American economics professor and lived in Buffalo, New York, where they raised their two children. After teaching economics for 15 years, her husband decided to become a minister. The family moved to Durham, North Carolina where Mr. Kraatz attended Duke University Divinity School, and Ms. Kraatz worked as an activity director in a nursing home. It was at this time that she also began to work as a freelance writer and editor.

Upon her husband's graduation from Duke, the family lived in North Carolina and then New York, where Mr. Kraatz served as a minister. During these years, Ms. Kraatz continued her work in nursing homes as an activity director and music therapist. When her editing and writing became a full-time career, she continued to be involved in nursing homes as a patient advocate and volunteer.

Ms. Kraatz and her husband now live in Ontario, Canada where he is a minister, and she continues her volunteer work in the U.S. and Canada as an advocate for nursing home residents and for the protection and improvement of their rights.